SUGAR BUSTERS!™

Shopper's Guide

Books published by The Ballantine Publishing Group are available at quantity discounts on bulk purchases for premium, educational, fund-raising, and special sales use. For details, please call 1-800-733-3000.

Published by Ballantine Books:

SUGAR BUSTERS!™: Cut Sugar to Trim Fat
SUGAR BUSTERS!™ Shopper's Guide

SUGAR BUSTERS!™

Shopper's Guide

H. Leighton Steward
Morrison C. Bethea, M.D.
Samuel S. Andrews, M.D.
Luis A. Balart, M.D.

BALLANTINE BOOKS • NEW YORK

A Ballantine Book
Published by The Ballantine Publishing Group
Copyright © 1999 by Sugar Busters, L.L.C.

www.randomhouse.com/BB/

Library of Congress Catalog Card Number: 98-96895

ISBN 0-345-43534-6

Manufactured in the United States of America

First Edition: January 1999

20 19 18 17 16 15 14 13 12

Table of Contents

Introduction

The authors of *Sugar Busters!: Cut Sugar to Trim Fat* have developed the *Sugar Busters! Shopper's Guide* to help you make better selections in your local grocery store, supermarket, and delicatessen. Many of you have voiced to us frustrations concerning which items are best for you. Grocery shopping is difficult. Advertising and labeling are often misleading and, at best, confusing. That is why we are including a section on reading labels. We, the authors of *Sugar Busters!*, know that our concept is valid, but, if you do not make correct choices regarding what you eat, it will not work for you. Therefore, we have developed this guide to help you succeed on *Sugar Busters!*

Sugar Busters! also is introducing its own products in categories where we feel there is the greatest demand. We have done this to ensure the availability of "legal " (or acceptable) *Sugar Busters!* products as well as to protect the integrity of our concept. Many of our products are available in your local area, but, if not, please ask your grocery store manager to contact Boudreaux Foods in New Orleans, Louisiana, who will make these products available in your local market.

The *Sugar Busters!* lifestyle is logical, practical, and reasonable. It does *not* involve weighing, measuring, or counting, but it does involve making better choices about what you eat, and it does involve moderation, especially in portion sizes. If you make healthy and nutritious choices and your servings of these choices are moderate, there is no need to worry about counting calories, which, in most instances, would be inaccurate and not even beneficial to what you are trying to achieve. *Sugar Busters!* is about lean and trimmed meats, high-fiber vegetables, whole grains, most fruits, and, if you choose, alcohol responsibly and in moderation.

Sugar Busters! is very careful and concerned about too much fat, especially saturated fat (animal as well as trans-fats, which are super-hydrogenated vegetable oils that are frequently used in commercial fast-food kitchens). On *Sugar Busters!* you generally will be eating forty percent (or slightly more) carbohydrates, thirty percent protein, and less than thirty percent fat, only ten percent of which should be saturated fat. These parameters are perfectly healthy and conform to those recommended by the American Heart Association. There are only a few common foods that you should avoid, such as potatoes, beets, corn, carrots, and some of the higher glycemic fruits, such as ripe bananas and raisins.

You will notice when shopping for *Sugar Busters!* items that your best choices are around the perimeter of the store rather than in the center, where the processed foods are. In making your choices, try to select those products that have as little refined sugar as possible, preferably no more than three grams of added refined sugar. Always remember that fresh is best, then frozen, and canned is often the least desirable. Different brands of the same food might vary considerably in the added ingredients. Therefore, initially reading labels until you are familiar with those items that are best for you will really help in cutting sugar.

Sugar Busters! also recommends exercise. Unfortunately, seventy percent of you do not and will not exercise, but you can still improve your weight and health by following the *Sugar Busters!* nutritional lifestyle.

What will *Sugar Busters!* do for you? It will help you achieve your ideal body weight (genetically predetermined), reduce your risks of diabetes and hypertension, and slow the aging of your blood vessels, as well as help prevent many other obesity-related health problems. If you are diabetic, *Sugar Busters!* will make it much easier to control your blood sugars. Those of you who suffer from hypoglycemia (low blood sugar) will also benefit from the *Sugar Busters!* lifestyle.

How is all of this achieved on *Sugar Busters!?* By eating in a healthy and nutritious fashion and by making better carbohydrate choices, you can go through the day with lower insulin levels. You cannot live without insulin, but you can live much better without too much insulin. Insulin, in addition to transporting glucose into cells for some of our energy needs, also makes you store sugar and fat as fat, prevents you from burning fat efficiently, and instructs your liver to produce additional amounts of cholesterol. Simply stated, higher than normal levels of insulin make us fat and flabby and our blood vessels age more quickly. This is something that we all would like to avoid, and the *Sugar Busters!* lifestyle will help you achieve this goal.

Try *Sugar Busters!* You will like it. You deserve to look and feel your best. It does not involve any costly supplements or additives but *only* involves making good, nutritious decisions about what you eat. This shopper's guide will help you get on your way. In addition, we have added a little Louisiana lagniappe ("something extra")—a section on how to eat out successfully on *Sugar Busters!*

Enjoy and *Bon Appétit!*

The Food Lists

What follows is a list of the various foods, grouped according to where they are generally found in the store. But first, here are a few overall tips on interpreting some things that might confuse you. For instance, when you pick up a can of boiled tomatoes and see that the listed ingredients are simply tomatoes and salt, yet the standard chart reads four grams of sugar, you should realize that tomatoes are really a fruit and, as such, must have their fructose content listed as sugar. This does not mean you should avoid boiled tomatoes! Remember, natural fructose is a good source of sugar and is not bad for you unless consumed in large quantities with other sugars during the same meal. The same goes for peanut butter, as long as there has been no sugar added.

Since cooking raises the glycemic index—or blood-sugar-elevating effect—

of carbohydrates, you can understand why it is better to replace most canned carbohydrates (except for green leafy vegetables) with the fresh, dried, or frozen variety.

When you prepare your dried beans, fresh vegetables, whole-grain pasta, or brown rice, do not overcook them. Instead, cook them al dente, or just a little bit firm. This will ensure a lower glycemic effect. Remember that your ancient ancestors actually ate their grains and vegetables completely raw—and obviously it worked just fine, otherwise we wouldn't be here today!

Finally, one last reminder so you will not have to count and measure: eat three platefuls a day with only appropriate snacks in between. A green salad on the side is all right. Do not cheat while you are trying to lose weight, but once you have achieved that goal, treat yourself occasionally to something that suits your fancy. But remember—too many treats will mean more fat on you!

The following lists will range from those containing some common brand names to simply a general statement, for example, that all unsweetened, no-sugar-added pickles are okay.

FRESH PRODUCE DEPARTMENT

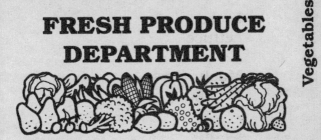

VEGETABLES
> Artichokes
> Arugula
> Asparagus
>
> Bean sprouts
> Bell pepper (red and green)
> Bok choy
> Broccoli
> Brussels sprouts
>
> Cabbage
> Cauliflower
> Celery
> Cucumber

Eggplant
Endive

Leeks
Lettuce

Mushrooms
Mustard greens

Okra
Onion—white, red, yellow

Peas
Pumpkin

Radicchio
Radishes

Sauerkraut
Snow peas
Spinach
Squash—yellow, butternut,
    spaghetti, acorn
String beans

Sweet potatoes/yams
(in moderation)

Tofu
Tomatoes
Turnip greens

Watercress

Zucchini

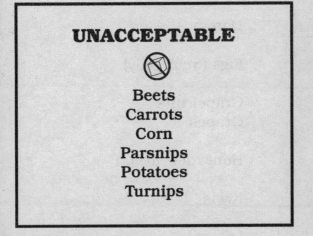

UNACCEPTABLE

Beets
Carrots
Corn
Parsnips
Potatoes
Turnips

FRUITS

Fruits

Apples
Apricots
Avocados

Blackberries
Blueberries
Boysenberries

Canteloupe
Cherries

Dates

Figs (fresh only)

Grapefruits
Grapes

Honeydew melon

Kiwis

Lemons

Limes

Mandarin oranges
Melons

Nectarines

Oranges

Peaches
Pears
Persimmons
Plums
Pomegranates

Raspberries

Satsumas
Strawberries

Tangerines

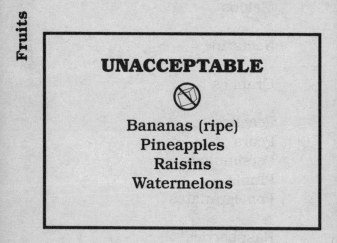

UNACCEPTABLE

Bananas (ripe)
Pineapples
Raisins
Watermelons

MEAT DEPARTMENT & REFRIGERATED ITEMS

Alligator
Antelope

Bacon (fat-free,
      not sugar cured)
Beef (lean and trimmed)

Canadian bacon
Chicken

Dove
Duck

Elk

Goose

Ham (if not sugar cured)

Hamburger: 85% lean or leaner

Lamb

Ostrich

Partridge
Pheasant
Pork

Quail

Rabbit

Sugar Busters!™ Chicken Cacciatore
Sugar Busters!™ Chili with Beans
Sugar Busters!™ Turkey & Sausage Gumbo

Turkey

Veal

Venison

UNACCEPTABLE

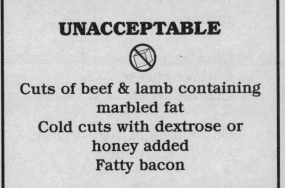

Cuts of beef & lamb containing
marbled fat
Cold cuts with dextrose or
honey added
Fatty bacon

DAIRY DEPARTMENT

Butter

Cheese
Cottage cheese
Cream

Dannon Light Yogurt with
    aspartame

Egg Beaters™
Eggs

Milk—2% or less fat preferred

Philadelphia® Cream Cheese
    (preferably light or low
    fat)

Sour cream (preferably light
    or low fat)

SEAFOOD DEPARTMENT

Alaskan pollock

Blue crab

Carp
Catfish
Clams (raw)
Cod
Crawfish

Dolphin
Dungeness crab

Eel

Grouper

Haddock
Halibut
Herring

King crab

Lobster

Mahi-Mahi
Monkfish
Mussels

Orange roughy
Oysters

Perch
Pike
Pompano

Redfish

Salmon
Scallops
Shrimp
Snails
Snapper
Snow crab
Sole

Tilapia
Trout
Tuna

Whitefish

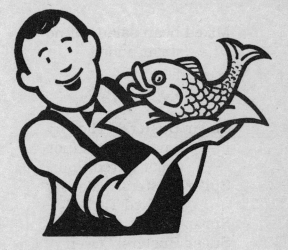

DELI

Cole Slaw, if no sugar added

Fruit salad, if no sugar added
and eaten as a meal

Green bean salad, if no sugar
added

Mixed bean salads, if no
sugar added

Roasted chicken

Sugar Busters!™ Hickory
Smoked Ham (not
sugar cured)
Sugar Busters!™ Hickory
Smoked Turkey
Sugar Busters!™ Lasagna
Sugar Busters!™ Oven
Roasted Turkey
Sugar Busters!™ Roast Beef

Tomato & cucumber salads,
etc., if no sugar added

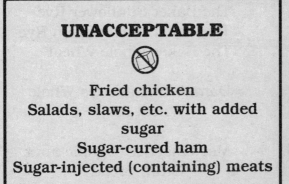

UNACCEPTABLE

Fried chicken
Salads, slaws, etc. with added
sugar
Sugar-cured ham
Sugar-injected (containing) meats

Deli

BAKERY/BREADS

ACCEPTABLE IN MODERATION

The Baker Pumpernickel
The Baker Sunflower Rye
The Baker Whole Grain Rye
The Baker Whole Wheat

Damascus Bakeries Whole
    Wheat Pita

Mestemacher Organic Four
    Grain Bread
Mestemacher Organic
    Sunflower Seed Bread
Mestemacher Organic Three
    Grain Bread
Mestemacher Whole Rye
    Bread

Sugar Busters!™ Whole Stone
    Ground Multigrain Loaf
    Bread

Sugar Busters!™ Stone
    Ground Whole Wheat
    Rustic Loaf Bread
Sugar Busters!™ Whole
    Wheat Baguettine
Sugar Busters!™ Whole
    Wheat Baguette
Sugar Busters!™ Whole Wheat
    Rounds
Sugar Busters!™ Whole Wheat
    Wraps

Toufayan Oat Bran Pita
Toufayan Whole Wheat Pita

Whole grain pumpernickel,
    100%
Whole grain rye, 100%
Wild's European Style
    Oatmeal Bread
Wild's Kommmisrot
Wild's Westphalian
    Pumpernickel
Wild's Whole Grain

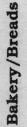

UNACCEPTABLE

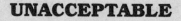

Breads that have sugars added
(including corn syrup, molasses,
etc.) or are not
whole grain breads

BEVERAGES

All diet sodas with aspartame

Caffeine-free diet colas
Crystal Light®

Diet colas
Diet ginger ale
Diet root beer
Diet tonic water

Lemonade (with aspartame)

No-sugar-added tea

Snapple diet drinks

TAB®

Beverages

35

SNACKS

ACCEPTABLE IN MODERATION

Finn Crisp®

Kavli® All Natural Whole
Grain Crispbread

Manischewitz whole wheat
Matzos

Ryvita® crackers (light & dark
rye)

Sugar Free Fat Free Jell-O
Gelatin/Pudding and
Pie Filling

Triscuit—deli-style rye
Triscuit—reduced fat

Wasa Fiber Rye
Wasa Hearty Rye
Wasa Light Rye
Wasa Multigrain

Snacks

Wasa Organic Rye
Whole grain wheat wafers

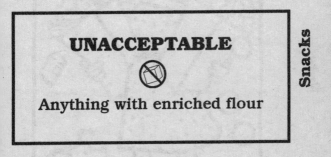

UNACCEPTABLE

Anything with enriched flour

NUTS

All nuts, without added
        sugar, honey, etc.
Almonds

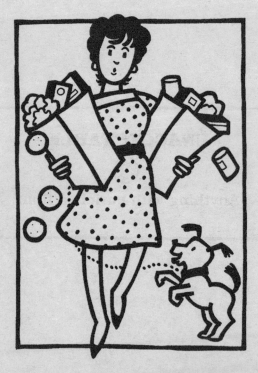

Brazil nuts

Cashews

Hazelnuts

Macadamia nuts

Peanuts, dry roasted
Pecans
Pistachios
Planters® Cashews, Almonds,
    and Macadamias—
    select mix
Planters® Dry Roasted
    Pistachios
Planters® Mixed Nuts
Planters® Select Mix
Pumpkin seeds

Sunflower kernels

Walnuts

BEANS

Black beans
Blackeye peas
Butter beans

Cannellini (white kidney
    beans)
Chickpeas (Garbanzo)

Green split peas

Kidney beans

Lentils

Navy beans

Pink beans

Soybeans

Wax beans

UNACCEPTABLE

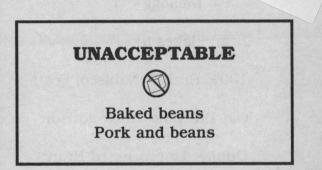

Baked beans
Pork and beans

ACCEPTABLE IN MODERATION

COLD CEREAL

All-Bran® Extra Fiber
(Kellogg's™)

Bran Flakes (Post)

100% Bran™ (Nabisco, Post)

Oat Bran (no sugar added)

Quaker Unprocessed Bran

Puffed Kashi Seven Grain &
Sesame

Shredded Wheat and Bran
(Post or Nabisco)

Uncle Sam's

Multi Grain Cheerios Plus
(General Mills)

Cereal

Hot Cereal

    Hodgson Mill® Oat Bran
    Hodgson Mill® Wheat Bran

    McCann's® Irish Oatmeal
    Mother's® 100% Natural Hot
        Cereal whole wheat
        rolled wheat

    Old World Bulgur Organic
        Wheat

Cereal

Quaker® Old-Fashioned
Oatmeal
Quaker® Instant Oatmeal
Regular Flavor
Quaker® Barley
Quaker® MultiGrain

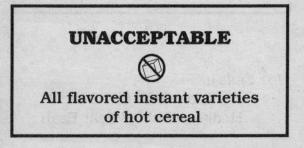

UNACCEPTABLE

All flavored instant varieties
of hot cereal

PANCAKE MIXES/FLOUR

Hodgson Mill® Buckwheat
Pancake Mix
Hodgson Mill® Rye Flour
Hodgson Mill® Whole Stone
Ground Flour

Pillsbury Whole Wheat Flour

Multigrain organic pancake
mix

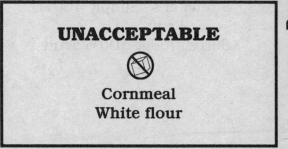

UNACCEPTABLE

Cornmeal
White flour

JAMS/JELLIES

ACCEPTABLE IN MODERATION

No-sugar-added jams and
jellies, in limited
amounts

Dickinson's® Purely Fruit™

Marie Sharp's All Natural
Papaya Jam, Orange,
Guava

Polaner® All Fruit®

St. Dalfour 100% Fruit
Smucker's® Simply 100%
Fruit®
Sorrell Ridge 100% Fruit

PEANUT BUTTER

No-sugar-added natural peanut butters

Smucker's® Natural

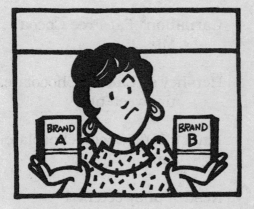

COCOA/CHOCOLATE

ACCEPTABLE IN MODERATION

All no-sugar-added baking chocolate

All chocolate with more than 60% cocoa, in limited amounts

Baker's® Unsweetened Baking Chocolate Squares

Carnation® Fat Free Cocoa Mix

Hershey's® Baking Chocolate, unsweetened

Lindt's 70% Cocoa chocolate bar

Nestlé® unsweetened

Nestlé® Choco-Bake, unsweetened

Swiss Miss® FatFree French Vanilla Hot Cocoa Mix

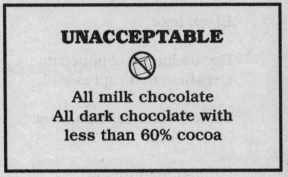

UNACCEPTABLE

All milk chocolate
All dark chocolate with
less than 60% cocoa

Cocoa/Chocolate

TEA/COFFEE

All decaffeinated coffee & tea

Black teas

Decaffeinated cappuccino
Decaffeinated espresso

Taster's Choice Regular or
Decaf

Limited amounts of
caffeinated types

JUICE

ACCEPTABLE IN MODERATION

Apple juice

Grape juice (no sugar added)
Grapefruit juice (fresh
squeezed or from
concentrate, no sugar
added)

Orange juice (fresh squeezed
or from concentrate, no
sugar added)

Tomato juice

Juice

SOUP

DRY SOUP
>Knorr®—Navy Bean, Lentil,
>Split Pea, Black Bean

>No-sugar-added types

>7 Bean & Barley Soup Mix

CANNED/CONDENSED SOUP
>All with no sugar added
>and/or white flour
>added

REFRIGERATED FRESH SOUP
>Sugar Busters!™ Black Bean
>Soup
>Sugar Busters!™ Lentil Soup
>Sugar Busters!™ 7 Bean
>Soup
>Sugar Busters!™ Tomato
>Basil Soup

UNACCEPTABLE

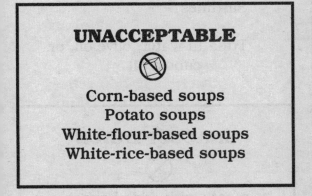

Corn-based soups
Potato soups
White-flour-based soups
White-rice-based soups

CANNED MEAT/FISH

All with no sugar added

Chicken in water

Salmon
Sardines

Tuna in water, olive oil, or
canola oil

UNACCEPTABLE

Meats with added sugar
Highly saturated fat meats

OLIVES/PICKLES/ GARNISHES

All with no sugar added

Capers
Cocktail onions

Dill pickles (with no sugar
    added)

Grape leaves

Olives, all

Pearl onions

Roasted peppers

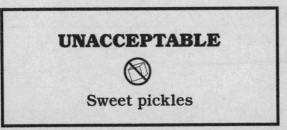

UNACCEPTABLE

Sweet pickles

CONDIMENTS

All no-sugar-added spices

Hot sauce, all, with no sugar
added

Mayonnaise (preferably light
or low fat with no sugar
added)

Mustards, all, with no sugar
added

Vinegar, all

CANNED FRUIT

All "legal" fruits with no sugar
added

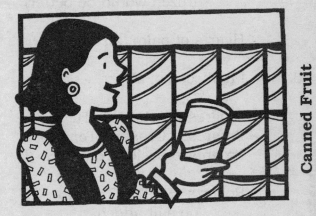

Canned Fruit

CANNED VEGETABLES

All "legal" vegetables with no
sugar added (fresh or
frozen would be better)

Hearts of palm, all

Mushrooms, all

Progresso Artichoke Hearts
Progresso Crushed Tomatoes
Progresso Peeled Tomatoes

Roberts' Big Red Tomatoes,
no salt added
Rotel Diced Tomatoes &
Green Chilies

Trappey's Beans—Black Eyed
Peas, Kidney, Pinto,
White Butter
Trappey's® Jalapeños

UNACCEPTABLE

Any prepared foods containing potatoes, corn, white rice, white flour, or significant amounts of carrots, white breading, or pasta

SPAGHETTI SAUCE

Classico®
Colavita Tomato Sauce,
London Style

Enrico's

Garden Valley Sundried
Tomato Salsa

Millina's

Sugar Busters!™ Pasta
Sauces

All others with no sugar
added

PASTA

ACCEPTABLE IN MODERATION

Bionature Whole Wheat Pasta

Capellini (angel-hair), in
    small amounts
Cuore Italiano Durum Wheat
    Semolina

De Boles® Whole Wheat Pasta

Eden Organic Golden Amber
    Durum Wheat

Hodgson Mill® Whole Wheat
    Fettucine
Hodgson Mill® Whole Wheat,
    Whole Grain Spaghetti
Hodgson Mill® Whole Wheat
    Spinach Spaghetti

Ravioli, cheese or meat filled

Stone ground whole wheat
    pastas

Sugar Busters!™ Stone Ground Whole Wheat pasta

Vitaspelt

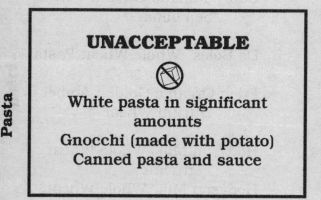

UNACCEPTABLE

White pasta in significant amounts
Gnocchi (made with potato)
Canned pasta and sauce

Pasta

GRAVY

All natural, no-sugar-added gravies

French's® or store brand gravy packets

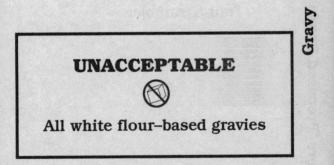

UNACCEPTABLE

All white flour–based gravies

BOX DINNERS/ PREPARED FOODS

Fantastic Foods® Semolina
Couscous

Hodgson Mill® Whole Wheat
Macaroni & Cheese

Tofu Burger
Tofu Scrambler

ETHNIC/SPECIALTY FOODS

Bamboo shoots
Bean threads (Chinese
    cellophane noodles)
Bok Choy

Fantastic Foods® Hummus

Guacamole

Matzo bread

Salsa
Snow peas
Soy sauce
Sugar Busters!™ Hummus
Sugar Busters!™ Salsa

Tabbouleh

Wakim's Food Hommus

Wakim's Food Babba Ghanouj
Water chestnuts
Whole wheat couscous
Whole wheat pita bread (see Bakery/Breads)
Whole wheat tortillas in moderation

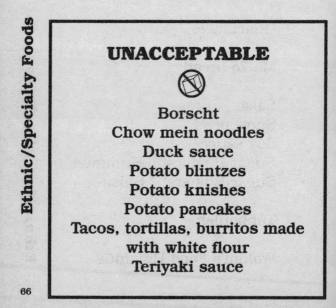

UNACCEPTABLE

Borscht
Chow mein noodles
Duck sauce
Potato blintzes
Potato knishes
Potato pancakes
Tacos, tortillas, burritos made with white flour
Teriyaki sauce

RICE

ACCEPTABLE IN MODERATION

Brown basmati rice
Brown rice (not instant)

Hadden House Extra Fancy
Cultivated Wild Rice

Kasha

Old World Pilaf

Texmati Basmati Brown Rice
Toasted almond pilaf

Wheat pilaf
Wild rice

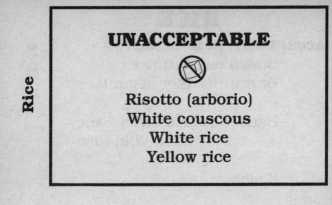

Rice

UNACCEPTABLE

Risotto (arborio)
White couscous
White rice
Yellow rice

SPICES

All with no added sugar

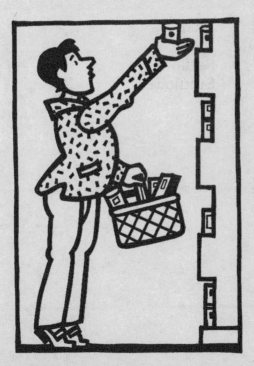

COOKING OIL

Canola
Corn

Olive

PAM®

Safflower
Sunflower

CAKE/FLOUR

ACCEPTABLE IN MODERATION
Stone ground whole wheat flours
but use artificial sweeteners
or very little sugar

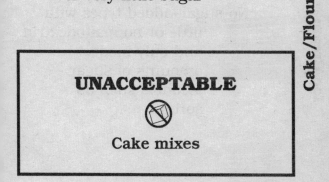

UNACCEPTABLE

Cake mixes

ICE CREAM

ACCEPTABLE IN MODERATION

Premium types with higher fat and lower sugar

No-sugar-added types with little or no maltodextrin and only modest amounts of sugar alcohols such as sorbitol

FROZEN FOOD

All "legal" vegetables
All using same criteria as
　　prepared foods

Boca Burgers

Garden Burgers
Gorton's® Grilled Fish Filets—
　　Lemon Pepper

Mrs. Paul's® Fish Fillets—
　　Lemon Pepper
Mrs. Paul's® Grilled Fish
　　Fillets
Mrs. Paul's® Grilled Salmon—
　　Creamy Dill

WINE

First choice, dry red wines
Second choice, dry white
wines

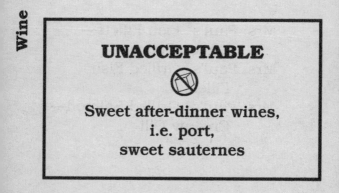

UNACCEPTABLE

Sweet after-dinner wines,
i.e. port,
sweet sauternes

Tips for
Lite-Weight Travel

Excess poundage, whether in your bags or around your middle, can make either business or personal travel a lot less comfortable. While many of us have figured out how to lighten our loads by choosing a few garments that mix and match well, most of us seem to be less creative when confronted with the menus placed before us in restaurants across the country. The fact that statistics show that we increase our risk for health problems as our body weight veers toward the obese (twenty percent or more overweight) should be incentive enough for us to learn how to make better choices now that the secret is out that it's primarily refined sugar and a handful of carbohydrates that cause the storage of most of our body fat.

Sugar can become body fat? Absolutely; it is explicitly stated in Arthur C. Guyton's *Textbook of Medical Physiology*. That's why we need to know how to bargain for alternatives when we are at the mercy of a menu and a waiter in places far from home.

The first, and usually the hardest, choice presents itself when a basket of warm, white, and probably fiberless bread is placed right under your nose. Beside it is usually a small bowl or a few pats of fresh butter. Bread smells great, you are hungry because it is mealtime, and your mouth begins to water. But first, you should ask for whole-grain or dark bread; they just might have it. Such substitutions are becoming commonplace, even in French-bread cities like New Orleans, Louisiana. It has been requested enough by the followers of the *Sugar Busters!* lifestyle that restaurants have responded favorably and have made healthier breads available.

Breads with a higher percentage of whole grains, while much better for your waistline, still should be eaten *in moderate quantities.* If restaurants just don't have acceptable bread, please resist the temptation to eat the highly refined white types. Making a bad decision at the beginning of a meal often turns into a "what-the-heck" attitude. You have already cheated, so, you might rationalize, you might as well order anything you want.

The list of appetizers can be quite limited

and occasionally all may be unacceptable. If none of them is totally acceptable, choose the one that has the least amount of "illegal" ingredients. Also, don't forget to check out the soups, since one might be an excellent substitution for an appetizer.

Ordering the main course is usually easier than trying to satisfy the white-bread or appetizer challenge. Fortunately, most restaurants will allow reasonable substitutions, and the easier you make it for them, the more likely they are to comply. To make it easy for the waiter, scan the vegetables offered with the various entrées and suggest that you would like the green beans from a different entrée instead of the mashed potatoes offered with your preferred entrée. It is difficult for a restaurant to deny you something already being prepared in its kitchen that day.

What do you do if the menu offers only low-fiber, blood-sugar-elevating carbohydrates like potatoes, corn, white rice, and white pasta? Don't give up! Good restaurants like to please you. Instead, ask for a grilled tomato or sautéed vegetables. If they cannot accommodate you, just eat the smallest amount of high-insulin-producing carbohydrates to get you through the meal.

If the sauce being served with your pork

chop is of a sweet variety, ask for it in a small dish on the side. That way, if your pork chop is cooked too dry, you can dab each bite of meat in the sauce instead of "pigging out" on a large amount of the sauce. As with substitutions for vegetables, check out other sauces being served and see if a low-sugar sauce is available.

Another tough decision comes when everyone at the table orders some sugary dessert and you don't want to sit there with an empty plate. If you have been moderate with your main meal, order some high-fiber berries like raspberries or strawberries topped with a little real cream and, if you must, sprinkle them with your favorite artificial sweetener. Or ask for a wedge of cheese, a cup of decaffeinated cappuccino, or, as the Europeans do, finish your meal with a green salad with a tasty sugar-free dressing.

If you are with a business guest and don't want to make your client feel self-conscious, simply order vanilla ice cream. While not ideal, most premium vanilla ice creams served in good restaurants contain only moderate amounts of sugar. If the restaurant doesn't have vanilla ice cream, you have at least tried to join your companion in a normal dessert and your guest won't think you are some strange antisocial individual. The worst thing you can do is end a great *Sugar Busters!* meal by giving in and eating a big sugary dessert and storing not only the sugar as body fat but increasing the problems that can occur when elevated insulin levels are present with any saturated fat you might have consumed with the rest of your meal.

Try these recommendations. You won't always succeed in getting what you wish, but if we all keep asking, more and better choices will appear. They are already showing up in cities outside New Orleans, and the expansion of choices should continue. Even better, more whole-grain, reduced-sugar products will be offered on a regular basis. It is very difficult to resist temptation when the choices are extremely limited or nonexistent, but again, keep asking and maybe someday even airline cuisine will change. Good luck and happy traveling and eating.

EXAMPLES OF NUTRITIONAL LABELS

Sugar Busters!
Acceptable

Sugar Busters!
Unacceptable

Nutrition Facts

Serving Size ⅓ cup (199g)
Servings Per Container 2½

Amount Per Serving

Calories 20   Calories from Fat 0

	% Daily Value*
Total Fat 0g	**0%**
Saturated Fat 0g	**0%**
Cholesterol 0mg	**0%**
Sodium 420mg	**17%**
Total Carbohydrate 3g	**1%**
Dietary Fiber 1g	**5%**
Sugars less than 1g	
Protein 2g	

Vitamin A 6%	•	Vitamin C 15%
Calcium 0%	•	Iron 2%

*Percent Daily Values are based on 2,000 calorie diet

INGREDIENTS: CUT GREEN ASPARAGUS, WATER, SALT

Nutrition Facts

Serving Size 2 cookies (33g)
Servings Per Container about 10

Amount Per Serving

Calories 150   Calories from Fat 60

	% Daily Value*
Total Fat 6g	**9%**
Saturated Fat 3.5g	**10%**
Cholesterol 35mg	**11%**
Sodium 110mg	**8%**
Total Carbohydrate 22g	**7%**
Dietary Fiber less than 1g	**4%**
Sugars 9g	
Protein 2g	

Vitamin A 4%	•	Vitamin C 0%
Calcium 2%	•	Iron 5%

*Percent Daily Values are based on a 2,000 calorie diet. Your daily values may be higher or lower depending on your calorie needs.

		Calories	2000	2,500
Total Fat	Less than		65g	80g
Sat. Fat	Less than		20g	25g
Cholesterol	Less than		300mg	300mg
Sodium	Less than		2,400mg	2,400mg
Total Carbohydrate			300g	375g
Dietary Fiber			25g	30g

Calories per gram:
Fat 9 • Carbohydrate 4 • Protein 4

INGREDIENTS: BUTTER, BLEACHED ENRICHED WHEAT FLOUR [CONTAINS BLEACHED WHEAT FLOUR, WHEAT FLOUR, NIACIN, REDUCED IRON, THIAMINE (VITAMIN B₁), MONONITRATES, RIBOFLAVIN (VITAMIN B₂), FOLIC ACID]; ROLLED OATS, SUGAR, FANCY MOLASSES, BROWN SUGAR, MILK, LEAVENING (BAKING POWDER, BAKING SODA); SALT, NATURAL FLAVOR

Reading Labels

Federal regulations require that food and beverage producers print certain "nutritional facts" on their product labels. Frequently, these facts are confusing and might even be misleading to the consumer. In an effort to help you better understand labeling and to make you a better *Sugar Busters!* shopper, we have included this section on reading labels.

Nutritional facts are based on a single recommended serving size. The information provided usually pertains to calories, total fats, carbohydrates, proteins, cholesterol, vitamins, minerals, and "other ingredients." We will discuss each one of these items separately so you can understand their significance.

Calories are a characteristic of each basic food source. There are approximately nine calories per gram of fat, seven calories per gram of alcohol, four calories per gram of carbohydrate, and four calories per gram of protein. Obviously, foods with a higher fat content per serving will have more calories than an equal amount of a carbohydrate or protein. Remember, calories are calculated from the basic components of the food product and do not have the importance of the following nutritional information.

Total fats are an important component of many food products. With the exception of meats, milk, and oils, fat grams should be very low—approximately one to three grams per serving. Lean, trimmed meats should have no more than five grams of fat per serving. Low-fat cheese should have no more than one to two grams of fat per serving. Two-percent milk should have slightly less than five grams per eight-ounce glass. Products with a normally high fat content, such as cooking oils, may contain as much as seven to nine grams of fat, but the largest percentage of this fat should be poly- or monounsaturated. These are the so-called good fats.

Many products contain trans-fats, which are vegetable oils to which additional hydrogen ions have been added during preparation. Trans-fats have the same effect on our bodies as saturated animal fats and, when possible, should always be avoided. New federal guidelines on nutritional information hopefully will require that trans-fats be listed on nutritional labels.

Trying to reduce your intake of unnecessary fats, especially saturated fats, is good, healthy, and recommended on *Sugar Busters!* However, we do need some fat for the proper functioning of our bodies. Removing all fat from your diet is not healthy. When it comes to fat, remember moderation. Equally as harmful to us as foods with too much fat are those that are advertised as low or no fat, which really means high sugar. Excessive amounts of added refined sugar will ultimately be converted to and stored in our bodies as fat.

Carbohydrates basically refer to all the sugar, either naturally occurring or added, in a particular food product. Fruits have a high content of fruit sugar (fructose), and milk products have a high content of milk sugar (lactose), but most carbohydrates are in the form of grains or starches and, as such, have very little simple sugars or "sugars." With the exception of fruits and dairy products, carbohydrate products, including grains and cereals, should contain no more than three grams of "sugars" per serving. A high "sugars" content—except in fruits and milk—is an important warning sign that the product is unacceptable on *Sugar Busters!* and probably has too much added refined sugar.

Fiber is an extremely important component of many carbohydrates. The higher the fiber content of a food product, the healthier it is for you. The incidence of colon cancer as well as some other medical problems is greatly reduced in those people eating a high-fiber diet. You should eat at least twenty grams of fiber daily. Green leafy vegetables are an excellent source of your daily fiber requirements.

Proteins may be derived from either plant or animal sources. Most of your protein will come from meat and dairy products, but grains and vegetables are also a good source. All balanced diets contain sufficient protein for your basic daily requirements.

Cholesterol is a component of most all meat and dairy products. You should avoid ingesting unnecessary cholesterol, but, in most people, diets containing several hundred milligrams of cholesterol a day are not harmful. Only forty percent of the ingested cholesterol is actually absorbed into our systems. But, when given a choice of different foods in a particular category, choose the ones with the lowest cholesterol content.

Vitamins and minerals are both important to the proper functioning of our bodies. A well-balanced diet as suggested by the authors of *Sugar Busters!* contains all the essential vitamins and minerals. A glass of freshly squeezed orange or grapefruit juice contains as much potassium as a banana. Most foods contain more than an adequate amount of *sodium.* You should be careful about adding additional salt when cooking or seasoning, especially if you have a heart or blood pressure problem. If you are concerned about your daily intake of sufficient vitamins and minerals, a good commercially available vitamin with minerals, such as Theragran-M and Centrum, more than ensures adequate daily intake of these substances.

Other ingredients are supplements and additives that processors have included in the preparation of their food products. These include maltodextrin, dextrose, xylol, maltose, malt, isomalt, sugar alcohol, high-fructose corn syrup, hydrolyzed starch, hydrolyzed rice starch, enriched flour, syrups, honey, and brown sugar. On the label, they are listed in order, from the largest to the smallest amount. Although some of these terms are not familiar to you, they all are disguised sugars. They have been added for the purpose of enhancing the taste or thickening the particular product. Their ultimate effect will be to raise your insulin levels and create more fat on your body. Sugar alcohols, which are often present in low-sugar diet ice creams, may cause gastrointestinal irritation and diarrhea. Although it is often difficult to avoid these additives altogether, every effort should be made to select those products that have as few and as little of these supplements as possible.

Beware of *enriched* bread, flour, and grain products. This means the manufacturer has stripped these foods of their natural fibers, minerals, vitamins, and other nutrients during processing. Enriching is an attempt to replace what nature already has provided but processing and refining have removed.

In summary, interpreting nutritional facts on food-product labels is not easy, but having a little knowledge about what this information means can make your shopping on *Sugar Busters!* much more successful.

The category you need to pay particular attention to is total fats, which should not exceed one to three grams per serving except in meat and milk products (which should not exceed five grams per serving) and cooking oils (which should predominantly be poly- or monounsaturated fats). Total carbohydrates should generally be between fifteen and twenty-five grams per serving, with sugars not to exceed three grams per serving except in fruit and dairy products. Remember to pick the product in the particular food category with the highest fiber content. This also applies to cholesterol, where those products in a particular food category with the lowest amount of total cholesterol are preferable. Other ingredients, in general, should be avoided as much as possible. This often can be achieved by selecting stone ground whole grains, fresh vegetables, and fruits. Cookies, cakes, pies, and most other low-fat and low-calorie items are full of the dreaded "other ingredients."

Your Personal Shopping List

As you become familiar with the acceptable brand-name products in your particular region of the country, add them to this guide to help you accomplish your grocery shopping more easily and quickly.

Vegetables

_____

_____

_____

_____

_____

_____

_____

_____

_____

_____

_____

_____

Fruits

_____

_____

_____

_____

_____

_____

_____

_____

_____

_____

_____

_____

Meat	Dairy
_____	_____
_____	_____
_____	_____
_____	_____
_____	_____
_____	_____
_____	_____
_____	_____
_____	_____
_____	_____
_____	_____
_____	_____

Seafood

_____

_____

_____

_____

_____

Deli

_____

_____

_____

_____

_____

Bakery/Breads

_____

_____

_____

_____

_____

Beverages

_____

_____

_____

_____

_____

Snacks

_____

_____

_____

_____

_____

Nuts

_____

_____

_____

_____

_____

Beans

_____

_____

_____

_____

_____

_____

Cereal (Cold/Hot)

_____

_____

_____

_____

_____

_____

Pancake Mixes/Flour   Jams/Jellies

_____   _____

_____   _____

_____   _____

Peanut Butter   Cocoa/Chocolate

_____   _____

_____   _____

_____   _____

Tea/Coffee   Juice

_____   _____

_____   _____

_____   _____

_____   _____

Soup (Dry/Canned)

_____

_____

Canned Meat/Fish

_____

_____

_____

Olives/Pickles/Garnishes/Condiments

_____

_____

_____

Canned Fruit

_____

_____

_____

Canned Vegetables

_____

_____

_____

Spaghetti Sauce

_____

_____

Gravy

_____

_____

Ethnic/
Specialty Foods

_____

_____

_____

_____

Pasta

_____

_____

_____

Box Dinners/
Prepared Foods

_____

_____

_____

Rice

_____

_____

_____

_____

Spices

Cooking Oil

_____

Cake/Flour   Ice Cream   Frozen Food

_____ _____ _____

_____ _____ _____

_____ _____ _____

Wine

Additional Items

_____ _____

_____ _____

_____

_____

_____

_____